GLAUCOMA COOKBOOK FOR BEGINNERS

Sight Savor: Nourishing Recipes And Expert Tips For Optimal Eye Health And Comfort-A Step By Step Guide For Novices

DR. JACE ZAYDEN

1

Table of Contents

Copyright © 2024, Dr. Jace Zayden

All Rights Reserved

No part of this publication may be reproduced, distributed, or transmitted in any form or by any means, including photocopying, recording, or other electronic or mechanical methods, without the prior written permission of the publisher, except in the case of brief quotations embodied in critical reviews and certain other noncommercial uses permitted by copyright law.

DISCLAIMER

The information provided in the book is intended for general informational purposes only. The content of this book should not be considered a substitute for professional medical advice, diagnosis, or treatment.

Readers are advised to consult with a qualified healthcare professional for medical advice tailored to their individual circumstances.

The author has made every effort to ensure that the information in this book is accurate and up-to-date at the time of publication. However, medical knowledge is constantly evolving, and new research may emerge that could impact the information presented. The author disclaims any responsibility for any adverse effects or consequences resulting from the use of the information provided in this book.

References or mentions of individuals, products, websites, organizations, or other names within this book are for informational purposes only and do not constitute an endorsement. The author has no affiliations with, and makes no endorsements of, any third-party entities mentioned. Readers are encouraged to conduct their own research and exercise their judgment when considering any external resources or recommendations.

The author and the publisher shall have neither liability nor responsibility to any person or entity with respect to any loss, damage, or injury caused or alleged to be caused directly or indirectly by the information contained in this book. Any reliance on the information within this book is at the reader's own risk.

By reading this book, the reader acknowledges and agrees to the terms of this disclaimer. If the reader does not agree with these terms, they should not use the information provided in this book.

ABOUT THIS BOOK

This "Glaucoma Cookbook" functions as an all-encompassing manual that underscores the critical significance of nutrition in the management of glaucoma, an enduring ocular disorder that, if untreated, may result in visual impairment. This book commences with a perceptive preface, furnishing readers with a fundamental comprehension of glaucoma and the consequences it entails. By exploring the significance of nutrition in the management of this condition, this cookbook enlightens readers about the direct influence that dietary decisions can exert on the health of the eyes.

The core of this book consists of an exhaustive examination of glaucoma-friendly foods and culinary methods that are specifically designed to promote ocular health. This cookbook conscientiously provides a variety of meal choices for every meal of the day, encompassing breakfast delicacies, midday staples, and dinner alternatives—everything included is intended to promote ocular health. By incorporating munchies, canapés, desserts, and beverages, the assortment of options suitable for individuals with glaucoma is increased, demonstrating how a comprehensive approach to nutrition can positively impact overall eye health.

Beyond its appetizing recipes, this "Glaucoma Cookbook" expands its audience by offering pragmatic advice on organizing meals to promote successful glaucoma management. To simplify the daily lives of individuals with glaucoma, this book additionally provides recommendations for conscientious purchasing. Additionally, it caters to unique events by including a section devoted to recipes tailored specifically for those occasions. In its capacity as a comprehensive resource, this cookbook expands its recommendations beyond nutrition to include lifestyle modifications that are instrumental in promoting overall ocular health.

By integrating knowledge of glaucoma management with culinary expertise, this cookbook transforms into an indispensable resource for those who wish to take preventative measures regarding their eye health. By its systematic arrangement of material, as well as its astute incorporation of recipes, advice, and recommendations for living a healthy life, this "Glaucoma Cookbook" establishes itself as an indispensable resource for individuals grappling with the complexities associated with glaucoma management via dietary and lifestyle modifications.

CHAPTER ONE

Introduction

A cluster of ocular disorders known as glaucoma causes optic nerve injury, which is commonly attributed to elevated intraocular pressure. Without intervention, it has the potential to result in irreversible vision impairment. Although medical interventions, such as glaucoma drops and surgery, are essential in the management of the condition, a healthy lifestyle, which includes consuming a balanced diet, can also be beneficial in preserving ocular health. A resource of its kind, The Glaucoma Cookbook, is intended to assist glaucoma patients in making well-informed dietary decisions that promote their ocular health and well-being as a whole.

Comprehension Of Glaucoma

To fully grasp the importance of adhering to a glaucoma-friendly diet, one must first acquire knowledge about the condition. Glaucoma is frequently referred to as the "silent thief of sight" due to its gradual progression and the fact that until the disease has reached its advanced phases, many individuals may remain asymptomatic. Damage to the optic nerve, which is accountable for transmitting visual information from the eye to the brain, causes peripheral vision loss over time.

Primarily, elevated intraocular pressure constitutes a risk factor for glaucoma. A disruption in the eye's constant fluid production and drainage can result in an increase in intraocular pressure, which can cause harm to the optic nerve. A multitude of glaucoma subtypes are recognized, with primary open-angle glaucoma being the most prevalent.

Early detection and treatment are of the utmost importance. Regular eye examinations are of the utmost importance, particularly for those who are at an increased risk, such as those aged 60 or above or those with a family history of glaucoma. Although surgical procedures and pharmaceutical interventions are designed to decrease intraocular pressure, a glaucoma-friendly diet may serve as a supplementary component and potentially impede the disease's advancement.

The Significance Of Nutrition In Glaucoma Management

It is becoming increasingly apparent that nutrition has a significant impact on ocular health, including conditions such as glaucoma, which is vital for maintaining overall health. Specific food items contain antioxidants, vitamins, and minerals that may aid in eye protection against oxidative stress and inflammation. These components hold significant importance in the management of glaucoma, as the optic nerve is prone to harm from these particular elements.

Existing research indicates that the optic nerve may be safeguarded by nutrients such as vitamin C, vitamin E, zinc, and omega-3 fatty acids; these nutrients may reduce the risk of developing glaucoma or delay its progression. Further, to ensure optimal eye health, it is crucial to manage conditions such as diabetes, which have the potential to worsen glaucoma, and maintain a healthy weight.

A balanced diet consisting of fruits, vegetables, whole cereals, lean proteins, and healthful fats is emphasized in The Glaucoma Cookbook. It promotes the restriction of processed foods, excessive carbohydrates, and saturated fats, all of which have been linked to inflammation and other health complications.

Diets Suitable For Glaucoma

As a result of their exceptional eye health benefits, specific foods are highlighted in the Glaucoma Cookbook. Antioxidants such as lutein and zeaxanthin, which are abundant in leafy green vegetables like kale and spinach, have been linked to a decreased likelihood of developing glaucoma. These nutrients have the potential to shield the eyes from ultraviolet radiation and other high-energy light waves.

The cookbook incorporates fish, particularly salmon and trout, which are rich in omega-3 fatty acids, due to their potential anti-inflammatory properties and ability to support healthy blood circulation. Nuts and seeds are also recommended, especially those that are rich in vitamin E, such as sunflower seeds and almonds.

Vibrant fruits and vegetables, such as bell peppers, oranges, and strawberries, are rich in antioxidants and vital vitamins. Vitamin C, which is particularly abundant in citrus fruits, may aid in the maintenance of healthy blood vessels in the eyes.

The cookbook additionally advocates for the inclusion of lean proteins, whole cereals, and legumes in the diet, thereby fostering a well-rounded and varied dietary regimen. Additionally, emphasis is placed on hydration, given that adequate water consumption is vital for sustaining overall health and assisting the body's innate detoxification mechanisms.

In summary, the Glaucoma Cookbook functions as an invaluable tool for individuals who are confronted with the difficulties associated with glaucoma management. Although not a replacement for medical intervention, incorporating a glaucoma-friendly diet into one's routine may enhance the overall health of individuals with glaucoma by supplementing conventional therapies. By acquiring knowledge about the condition, acknowledging the significance of nutrition, and integrating glaucoma-friendly foods into their daily diets, individuals can adopt a proactive stance in favor of their visual well-being and potentially impede the advancement of this perilous ailment.

Techniques Of Preparation For Glaucoma-Friendly Meals

A group of eye conditions known as glaucoma, which causes injury to the optic nerve, necessitates meticulous dietary considerations to promote eye health.

This Glaucoma Cookbook serves as a vital resource for the management of this condition, providing individualized recipes that incorporate ingredients that enhance the health of the eyes. Conversely, the cookery methods utilized to safeguard the nutritional integrity of these components are of equivalent significance.

Steaming and simmering are recognized as exceptional methods for preparing dishes that are suitable for individuals with glaucoma. These techniques preserve vital nutrients while preventing the addition of excessive lipids. Vegetables such as kale and spinach that are steamed retain their antioxidant content, including lutein and zeaxanthin, which are recognized for their ability to support eye health. Boiling grains such as quinoa or brown rice preserve their nutritional profile and provide a substantial foundation for recipes suitable for individuals with glaucoma.

The integration of these methodologies during the culinary procedure not only amplifies the nutritional composition of dishes but also facilitates their digestion. By prioritizing the adoption of healthier culinary techniques, individuals diagnosed with glaucoma can actively contribute to the maintenance of optimal ocular health via their dietary choices.

CHAPTER TWO

Delights For Eye Health At Breakfast

In addition to serving as a nourishing start to the day, a glaucoma-friendly breakfast should also contain vital nutrients that promote eye health. Because the initial meal of the day establishes the tone for overall health, individuals with glaucoma must ensure that they incorporate mindful decisions into their morning regimen.

A fundamental component of a breakfast that is suitable for individuals with glaucoma is the inclusion of foods that are abundant in antioxidants such as zeaxanthin and lutein, in addition to vitamins A, C, and E. A smoothie containing a hint of citrus, spinach, and fruit delivers a potent dose of these nutrients. Chia seeds, which are rich in omega-3 fatty acids, can be used as a garnish to enhance visual appeal and provide a contrast in texture.

Consider incorporating whole grain alternatives, such as oatmeal or whole wheat toast, into your glaucoma-aware breakfast routine. They facilitate the sustained discharge of energy and improve blood circulation, both of which are essential for the preservation of eye health. Adding sliced avocados, which are rich in nutrients such as lutein, to these dishes enhances their flavor and provides visual benefits.

Egg yolks, in particular, are an excellent source of zeaxanthin and lutein, two nutrients that are beneficial for glaucoma patients to include in their breakfast. By selecting poached or simmered eggs instead of frying eggs, one can preserve their nutritional value while avoiding the addition of excessive lipids.

Favorites For Lunchtime With Glaucoma

Lunch provides a vital opportunity to nourish the eyes and replenish the body, thus justifying its inclusion in a diet that is conducive to glaucoma. It is crucial to incorporate foods that are abundant in antioxidants, vitamins, and minerals, all of which are beneficial for the health of the eyes.

Greens that are leafy atrophy are the main course during brunch. Arugula, spinach, and kale comprise a salad that is rich in numerous nutrients, such as lutein and zeaxanthin. Carrots and bell peppers are two colorful vegetables that can be used to increase their antioxidant content. Incorporating a light vinaigrette crafted from olive oil, which is renowned for its anti-inflammatory attributes, concludes a revitalizing and aesthetically pleasing brunch.

For a protein-rich supper, fish, especially those rich in omega-3 fatty acids such as trout or salmon, can be grilled or roasted. Omega-3 fatty acids have been identified as contributors to optic nerve maintenance and overall eye health. Fish accompanied by brown rice or quinoa constitutes a well-balanced meal that promotes glaucoma management and overall health.

Incorporating legumes such as chickpeas or lentils into a luncheon stew or curry presents a flavorful and nutrient-dense alternative for vegetarians. Zinc, which is abundant in legumes, has been linked to a decreased risk of developing glaucoma.

Dinner Selections That Promote Eye Health

The last opportunity of the day to nourish the eyes and body with a well-balanced, glaucoma-aware meal is at dinner. Incorporating culinary methods that maintain the nutritional value of ingredients while selecting those that support eye health is crucial when preparing a meal that caters to the dietary requirements of individuals with glaucoma.

An entrée suitable for individuals with glaucoma primarily consists of grilled vegetables and lean proteins. In addition to possessing a robust antioxidant profile, vegetables such as Brussels sprouts, asparagus, and broccoli impart a gratifying texture when grilled.

When accompanied by grilled poultry or tofu, they offer a sustainable source of protein that is low in saturated lipids.

By integrating whole cereals such as bulgur or quinoa into dinner recipes, one can enhance the nutritional value. Zinc, which is present in these cereals, is among the vital vitamins and minerals that promote eye health. Stir-frying an assortment of vibrant vegetables alongside tofu or shellfish presents a time-efficient and wholesome alternative for supper.

Herbs and seasonings can be utilized in abundance to augment the taste of banquets suitable for individuals with glaucoma while maintaining their health. Due to its anti-inflammatory characteristics, turmeric may be incorporated into condiments or preparations. Ginger and garlic not only enhance the flavor of food but also promote general health.

In conclusion, a Glaucoma Cookbook offers guidance to individuals with glaucoma towards a holistic approach to preparing and consuming, surpassing the mere provision of recipes. By employing particular culinary methodologies and choosing components abundant in eye-beneficial nutrients, every meal assumes the role of a proactive measure toward bolstering general eye well-being and efficiently managing glaucoma.

CHAPTER THREE

Glaucoma Snacks And Appetizers

For those afflicted with glaucoma, it is vital to adhere to a diet designed to promote eye health. Snacks and appetizers are substantial contributors to the attainment of this objective, as they provide a chance to integrate eye-healthy nutrients into one's diet while simultaneously gratifying desires. The objective of a Glaucoma Cookbook devoted to appetizers and refreshments is to furnish not only delectable alternatives but also vital nutrients that promote ocular health.

Nuts and seeds are exceptionally beneficial treats for individuals with glaucoma. For instance, almonds, walnuts, and chia seeds are rich in vitamin E and omega-3 fatty acids, which are recognized for their potential to safeguard the optic nerve. These ingredients, when combined to make a trail mix, guarantee a satiating and crispy refreshment that also supports eye health.

Combining vegetable skewers with hummus or yogurt-based condiments presents a pleasurable method of augmenting one's consumption of antioxidants. Carrots, bell peppers, and celery are excellent sources of vitamin C and beta-carotene, both of which are beneficial to the eyes' overall health. The addition of protein and fiber to hummus made from chickpeas makes it a nutritious option for those with glaucoma.

Additionally, consuming seafood can be advantageous. Tuna or salmon may be incorporated into micro fish cakes or pastries. Omega-3 fatty acids, which are abundant in these species, possess anti-inflammatory properties that could potentially aid in the reduction of intraocular pressure that is linked to glaucoma.

For individuals with glaucoma, it may be prudent to select whole-grain wafers or rice cakes. Whole grains are a valuable source of nutrients, including zinc and niacin, which play a significant role in promoting eye health. By incorporating avocado, which is rich in lutein and zeaxanthin, the eye-enhancing properties of the food are further intensified.

Sweet Treats And Desserts Containing Eye-Enhancing Ingredients

Desserts and delectable delights can remain a component of a diet suitable for individuals with glaucoma if prepared with appropriate ingredients. By integrating elements recognized for their ability to enhance ocular well-being, commonplace delights can be transformed into nutritional powerhouses.

Blueberries and strawberries, among other berries, are abundant in anthocyanins, which are antioxidants that potentially promote eye health. Berry parfait containing Greek yogurt not only fulfills the desire for sweetness but also imparts protein and probiotics, thereby making a positive contribution to one's overall health.

In moderation, dark chocolate can be a delectable addition to a confection that is suitable for those with glaucoma. The flavonoids present in dark chocolate may assist in increasing blood flow to the eyes. Producing chocolate-coated fruits, such as cherries or bananas, presents a confectionery indulgence that may also have anti-aging properties.

By incorporating nuts, such as almonds and walnuts, into delicacies, omega-3 fatty acids and vitamin E are added in addition to texture. Individuals with glaucoma can indulge in gratifying and nourishing treats such as almond-studded oat bars or nut-infused energy balls.

Desserts made from avocado offer a silky consistency and supply lutein and zeaxanthin, which are critical nutrients for maintaining healthy eyes. Optimistic dessert choices for individuals with glaucoma may include avocado chocolate mousse or a pleasant sorbet composed of avocado and citrus.

Beverages That Promote Eye Health

It is vital for overall health, including eye health, to maintain adequate hydration. The objective of the beverages segment in A Glaucoma Cookbook is to offer invigorating choices that not only satiate desire but also aid in the management of glaucoma.

Catechins, which are abundant in green tea, are antioxidants that may be beneficial for individuals with glaucoma. Antioxidants have the potential to safeguard the eyes against oxidative stress. In addition to enhancing the flavor, the inclusion of a dash of citrus (such as lemon or orange) provides an additional source of vitamin C.

Smoothies are multifunctional and provide an inventive method to integrate ingredients that enhance vision. Supplementing with leafy greens such as kale, spinach, or Swiss chard offers a dietary source of zeaxanthin and lutein.

The incorporation of fruits, such as kiwis or mangoes, not only improves the flavor but also provides vital micronutrients.

Carrot juice is a time-honored remedy for enhancing eye health. A precursor to vitamin A, carrots are an excellent source of beta-carotene, an essential nutrient for maintaining healthy eyesight. Carrot juice that has been lightly blended with turmeric or ginger can be enhanced in flavor and provide anti-inflammatory properties.

Infusing water with cucumber segments or mint serves the dual purpose of providing hydration and introducing a refreshing element. Maintaining proper hydration is critical for preserving eye health and potentially aids in the regulation of intraocular pressure.

The Management Of Glaucoma Via Meal Planning

Meal planning is an essential component of successful glaucoma management as it guarantees the consumption of essential nutrients while regulating variables that could potentially affect eye health. A Glaucoma Cookbook devoted to meal preparation offers individuals coping with this condition guidance on how to prepare nutritious and well-balanced meals.

It is crucial to include an assortment of vibrant vegetables in a meal plan that is suitable for individuals with glaucoma. Vegetables such as broccoli, spinach, and kale are abundant in nutrients and antioxidants that promote eye health. Vegetable-based casseroles, stir-fries, and salads are all excellent methods to incorporate these vital ingredients.

Incorporating lean proteins, including poultry, fish, and legumes, into one's diet is crucial for the provision of omega-3 fatty acids and essential amino acids. Salmon that has been grilled, lentil stew, or a quinoa salad containing broiled chicken is all protein-rich meals that support glaucoma management objectives.

To improve the nutritional value of dishes, refined cereals ought to be substituted with whole grains. As substitutes, brown rice, quinoa, and whole-grain pasta may be utilized. The zinc, niacin, and fiber content of these grains all contribute to the maintenance of eye health.

To effectively manage glaucoma, it is vital to restrict sodium consumption, as elevated sodium levels can cause an increase in intraocular pressure. A fundamental component of a meal plan suitable for individuals with glaucoma is the substitution of sodium with fresh herbs, seasonings, and other methods of flavor enhancement.

In summary, a Glaucoma Cookbook that provides comprehensive guidance on meal planning, munchies, desserts, and beverages serves as an invaluable resource for those coping with this condition. By integrating ocular-enhancing components and adhering to a nutritionally balanced regimen, these recipes not only promote holistic health but also contribute to the eye's welfare, thereby augmenting the quality of life for individuals afflicted with glaucoma.

CHAPTER FOUR

Everyday Strategies For Managing Vision

Glaucoma presents individuals with particular difficulties, but a deliberate and strategic approach to daily activities—such as cooking, purchasing, and lifestyle decisions—can substantially improve the standard of living for those afflicted. This investigation examines three essential facets of glaucoma management: Strategies for Purchasing with Glaucoma in Consideration, Recipes for Special Occasions, and Lifestyle Modifications for Comprehensive Eye Care.

Shopping Advice To Keep Glaucoma In Mind

Grocery store aisles can be a formidable obstacle for those afflicted with glaucoma, an eye condition marked by elevated intraocular pressure that may result in optic nerve impairment and visual impairment. However, by implementing some strategic planning, the act of purchasing can be transformed into a more enjoyable and manageable experience.

1. Before visiting the store, compile an exhaustive inventory of the items that you require. Product categorization facilitates product discovery within the store. Make use of smartphone applications that provide voice-guided lists or magnification capabilities to accommodate individuals with visual impairments.

2. Make a conscious decision and visit supermarkets that have sufficient illumination. Adequate lighting conditions improve visibility, thereby facilitating label reading and ensuring safe navigation within the store. Crawl-free zones should be avoided, as they can heighten the likelihood of unintended collisions.

3. Investigate Online Shopping: Acknowledge the ease and utility of purchasing groceries online. This service is now provided by numerous retailers, enabling customers to shop from the convenience of their residences. Frequently,

online marketplaces feature intuitive interfaces and exhaustive product descriptions.

4. Deciding to purchase pre-packaged and labeled foods can streamline the process of grocery purchasing. Labeled packaging that is conspicuously marked with large, high-contrast fonts promotes comprehension. Consider purchasing products that are braille labeled or that are designed specifically for users with visual impairments.

5. Requesting Assistance: It is impolite to remain silent when seeking assistance. In general, store personnel exhibit a willingness to aid patrons, particularly those who have particular requirements. Personal purchasing services are provided by several grocery stores to customers with disabilities.

6. Employ Magnifying Instruments: To read labels and prices, carry a portable magnifier or utilize the magnification feature on your smartphone. When purchasing, these resources

can be indispensable in ensuring that you make well-informed decisions.

7. Be Aware of Expiration Dates: To ensure the freshness of products, check their expiration dates and refrain from purchasing items that may not be consumed before their expiration. To discern these dates, one may utilize a smartphone application equipped with optical character recognition (OCR) capabilities or a magnifying glass.

Occasion-Specific Recipes

Glaucoma management requires a well-balanced diet, but this does not have to compromise flavor or enjoyment. These glaucoma-friendly recipes guarantee that special occasions, be they intimate gatherings or festive celebrations, are not only delectable but also beneficial to eye health.

1. Walnut and Spinach Salad:

• Fresh spinach, hazelnuts, cherry tomatoes, olive oil, and balsamic vinegar are the ingredients.

• Approach: Combine arugula, cherry tomatoes that have been halved, and minced walnuts. Incorporate olive oil and balsamic vinegar into the salad to enhance its flavor and nutritional value.

2. Salmon marinated in lemon herb oil and grilled:

Salmon fillets, lemon juice, olive oil, garlic, fresh herbs (thyme, rosemary), salt, and pepper are the ingredients.

• Approach: Plunge salmon fillets in an emulsion composed of fresh herbs, minced garlic, lemon juice, and olive oil. Grill until thoroughly cooked. Salmon's high omega-3 fatty acid content is beneficial to eye health.

3. Stir-fried quinoa and Vegetables:

• Quinoa, assorted vegetables (carrots, bell peppers, and broccoli), soy sauce, ginger, and garlic are the ingredients.

Cook the quinoa according to the instructions on the package. An assortment of vibrant vegetables is stir-fried with soy sauce, garlic, and ginger. Combine with quinoa to create an aesthetically pleasing and nourishing dish.

4. The Blueberry Parfait is:

Greek yogurt, organic blueberries, honey, and granola are the ingredients.

• Procedure: Greek yogurt, granola, and fresh blueberries are layered. Honey can be used to impart flavor. Blueberries comprise antioxidants that promote the health of the eyes.

5. Grilled Mango Salsa Chicken:

Ingredients: mango salsa (comprising mango, red onion, cilantro, and lime juice), grilled chicken breast.

• Technique: Saturate seared chicken with mango salsa prepared in-house. Mangoes are rich in vitamins A and C, both of which are critical for eye health.

The ingredients utilized in these recipes are concentrated in antioxidants, vitamins, and minerals, all of which are beneficial for the eye. Please ensure that you consult a healthcare professional or nutritionist to verify that these recipes are suitable for your specific dietary requirements.

Changes In Lifestyle For General Eye Care

In addition to dietary modifications, the incorporation of lifestyle adjustments can make a substantial impact on the holistic ocular health of glaucoma patients. By integrating these practices into one's daily regimen, one can potentially promote eye health and impede the advancement of the condition.

1. Consistent Ocular Examinations: Establish a routine schedule for eye examinations with an ophthalmologist to track the advancement of glaucoma and modify your treatment regimen as required.

2. Chronic tension has the potential to impact intraocular pressure. Participate in stress-relieving practices such as yoga, meditation, or deep breathing exercises to enhance one's overall health.

3. Maintaining proper hydration is critical for the preservation of eye health. Throughout the day, consume copious amounts of water to maintain appropriate fluid balance in the eyes.

4. Prevent UV Interruption: When venturing outdoors, don sunglasses that offer UV protection to shield your eyes. Extended UV radiation exposure could potentially accelerate the development of glaucoma.

5. Consistent Physical Activity: Incorporate regular, moderate exercise into your routine. Physical activity enhances circulation and blood flow, which is advantageous for eye health as a whole.

6. A sufficient amount of sleep should be obtained each night. A sufficient amount of high-quality

sleep is essential for the overall health of the body, including the eyes.

7. Observe Side Effects of Medication: Certain medications may affect eye health. When considering medication usage for conditions other than glaucoma, it is advisable to consult your healthcare provider regarding potential adverse effects.

8. Cessation of smoking has been associated with an elevated likelihood of developing glaucoma and worsening its advancement. Eliminating tobacco use may result in improved ocular health.

By adopting these modifications to your way of life and incorporating glaucoma-friendly recipes into your diet, you can take an active role in managing your condition and improving your overall health. It is imperative to seek personalized advice and guidance tailored to one's specific requirements from the healthcare team.

Conclusion

In summary, the Glaucoma Cookbook functions as an invaluable tool for individuals who are confronted with the dietary obstacles that are inherent to glaucoma. Using its meticulously designed recipes and astute nutritional counsel, the cookbook not only discusses the significance of adopting a health-conscious way of life in the management of glaucoma but also advocates for holistic wellness.

The cookbook's prioritization of foods abundant in antioxidants, vitamins, and minerals is consistent with scientific findings that propose specific nutrients might contribute to ocular health support and potentially impede the advancement of glaucoma. By incorporating components recognized for their beneficial effects on intraocular pressure and general ocular well-being, the cookbook's pertinence in the realm of glaucoma management is reinforced.

Furthermore, the Glaucoma Cookbook surpasses basic dietary suggestions by integrating a comprehensive methodology that takes into account the interdependence of lifestyle, nutrition, and ocular well-being. It promotes the adoption of practices that are beneficial to one's overall health, thereby encouraging readers to experience a positive influence on their glaucoma voyage.

Fundamentally, this cookbook not only offers a wide selection of delectable and ocular health-conscious recipes but also encourages readers to adopt an informed stance regarding their vision. Utilizing its exhaustive nature, the Glaucoma Cookbook serves as an indispensable resource for individuals aiming to improve their overall health by making conscientious and nourishing dietary selections.

THE END

www.ingramcontent.com/pod-product-compliance
Lightning Source LLC
Chambersburg PA
CBHW060817260726
48660CB00002B/998